LIVING IN BALANCE

"This gem of a book goes where others have not gone, offering practical emotional, physical, psychological, and most importantly, spiritual clues to aid in recovery. Using meditations as the basis for this ninety-day journey, this book offers keys to recovery and is a significant contribution to the field. It can (and should) be used for daily reflections at rehabilitation centers, by individuals and groups in early recovery, and serve as an essential tool even for those with longer-term recovery. It is a wonderful compendium in one volume of what you might otherwise find spread out in several books, brought together in a single, coherent, useful, practical, step-by-step guidebook. I highly recommend it to colleagues, treatment programs, and those on the path of recovery."

David J. Powell, Ph.D.
President, International Center for Health Concerns
East Granby, CT

"Recovery is a lifelong journey about understanding and accepting who we are. This new book emphasizes that love and its healing power are at the center of this journey. As a woman, and for other women in recovery, this book of daily meditations will help ground each day with profound spiritual depth. Although wisdom and patience usually come with age, this book offers its healing message in a simplistic form that is easy to absorb yet powerful if taken seriously as a daily practice. Congratulations to the author for this beautiful offering."

Wendee Wechsberg, Ph.D.
Senior Director,
Substance Abuse Treatment Evaluations and Interventions
RTI International
Research Triangle Park, NC

"Dr. Hoffman brilliantly brings the deserved emphasis to holistically living in balance in this empathetic guide. Its depth and simplicity make for a novel and highly useful companion in the treatment of addiction that practitioners and other readers should enjoy."

ERIC T. MOOLCHAN, M.D.
Addiction Research Scientist and former Medical Director
ADAPT Multi-Modality Treatment Program
Washington D.C.

"A successful book and a useful tool for our daily lives and for addicts in recovery."

MIN ZHAO, M.D., PH.D.
Professor of Psychiatry, Shanghai Mental Health Center
Shanghai Jiao Tong University School of Medicine
Shanghai, China

"*Living in Balance: 90 Meditations for Recovery from Addiction* reflects both the author's professional background in the addiction field as well as his personal family experiences. The book illustrates the many factors of addiction, including the genetics contributing to the development of that chronic relapsing disorder. *Living in Balance* points out clearly that recovery requires not only the individual's decision to stop using and the irreplaceable support of family, but also that a supportive environment is critical for change. Its ninety meditations inform readers that time itself is an important issue and what seems like small steps to some might be very big ones for others!"

GABRIELE FISCHER, M.D.
Medical Director, Addiction Clinic
Medical University of Vienna, Austria

"Dr. Hoffman's personal touch and deep understanding of addiction serve as a strong base for the steps outlined in *Living in Balance: 90 Meditations for Recovery from Addiction.* Surely people suffering from addictions will find this book very useful. Its simple presentation makes the messages and meditations stronger for many."

ELI LAWENTAL, D.S.W.
Director, Haifa Drug Abuse Treatment Center
Department Head of Social Work
Tel-Hai College, Haifa, Israel

"This book takes the reader on a journey through the concepts of meditation to the depths of recovery and finding joy in their world through self-empowerment. Fantastic!"

CYNTHIA MORENO TUOHY
Executive Director, NAADAC, the Association for
Addiction Professionals
Washington D.C.

"'The journey of a thousand miles begins with a single step,' the Chinese sage Lao Tzu remarked some 1,500 years ago. The journey of recovery, too, begins in the same way. Challenges lie ahead to be sure. Thankfully, Dr. Jeff Hoffman has penned a simple and elegant volume of reflections and meditations to accompany you along the way. Taken day by day, they nourish the soul and help build a foundation for living life in balance."

SCOTT D. MILLER, PH.D.
Director, International Center for Clinical Excellence
Chicago, IL

"*Living in Balance: 90 Meditations for Recovery from Addiction* is a warm companion on the way-seeking path. Read it each morning, savor it throughout the day, and allow it to inspire a mindful attitude in this precious life. Dr. Hoffman offers wisdom, daily affirmations, and practical advice on how to fill the holes in our soul—those longings we tried to numb with drugs, alcohol, or other compulsive acts. Read these ninety meditations in ninety days and realize a new strength and a new hope to living free from addiction."

Thérèse Jacobs-Stewart
St. Paul, MN
Author of Mindfulness and the 12 Steps:
Living Recovery in the Present Moment

HAZELDEN MEDITATIONS

LIVING IN BALANCE

90 MEDITATIONS FOR RECOVERY FROM ADDICTION

JEFFREY A. HOFFMAN, PH.D.

HAZELDEN®

Hazelden
Center City, Minnesota 55012
hazelden.org

Library of Congress Cataloging-in-Publication Data

Hoffman, Jeffrey A., 1955–
Living in balance : 90 meditations for recovery from addiction / Jeffrey A. Hoffman.
p. cm.
Includes index.
ISBN 978-1-61649-087-4 (softcover)
1. Substance abuse—Psychological aspects. 2. Meditation. 3. Affirmations. 4. Drug addicts—Rehabilitation. 5. Alcoholics—Rehabilitation. I. Title.
HV4998.H64 2011
616.86'06—dc22

2010037817

Editor's note
Alcoholics Anonymous, AA, and the Big Book are registered trademarks of Alcoholics Anonymous World Services, Inc.

15 14 13 12 11 1 2 3 4 5 6

Cover and interior design by David Spohn
Cover illustration by Nicholas Wilton
Typesetting by BookMobile Design and Publishing Services

In memory of my dearest sister Debbie—my favorite dance partner—who struggled and turned the darkness of addiction into light, and to her two beloved children: Matthew and Jamie

ACKNOWLEDGMENTS

Special thanks to my awesome editor, coach, and friend, Richard Solly, who with his depth of knowledge and experience of recovery gave this little book just the right needed touch.

FOREWORD

BY EDWARD TEYBER, PH.D.

It's very hard to make deep changes that transform how we live. It is so promising when, after struggling with an addiction, we truly grasp that something is terribly wrong and make a personal commitment to recovery. But this commitment—and then maintaining sustained engagement in the healing process—is hard to achieve. For most, it does not come easily. We will need help if we are to succeed. Painful and complex problems originally led us into our addictions. There has been plenty of heartache for those who cared and tried to help us along the way. It's difficult to hold to our resolve when familiar patterns and pain emerge yet again and threaten to overwhelm us. Thankfully, *Living in Balance: 90 Meditations for Recovery from Addiction* offers real help. This book provides the practical help that can make a difference in our everyday lives and help us sustain our goal of recovery—"one day at a time."

Dr. Jeff Hoffman is an internationally acclaimed expert on addiction and recovery. He knows as much about this work as anyone. Dr. Hoffman and I have been close friends since we were teenagers and have been colleagues for decades. I think he learned the most important things about intervention, treatment, and recovery from growing up with the heartbreak of having deeply loving parents and family members who struggled long and mightily with addiction. Perhaps that's why you'll find the simple guidelines he offers here so practical, useful, and above all, real. You'll recognize immediately that he knows what he's writing about. He shares his deep understanding with such compassion and respect. You will find no unwanted judgments here—no subtle criticism or control. Instead, Dr. Hoffman is offering something of what every good parent or family member offers to a child or a skilled therapist to a client: genuine understanding and encouragement to address problems directly rather than deny or avoid them. His book offers realistic guidelines, not false reassurances or superficial solutions that only put rose-colored glasses on serious problems.

So how does this book help? Dr. Hoffman teaches how to begin a simple, daily meditation practice that provides a safe harbor from the waves that can overtake us, make us fall back on familiar but problematic patterns, and threaten to take us down. He uses meditation as part of a life plan, a road map that offers an invaluable guide to those who choose to undertake this recovery journey.

When I first met Dr. Hoffman, he was just nineteen years old. He could always help me (as he did with many others over the decades) with whatever big or small problem I brought to him. He did so by using the same compassion, straight talk, and good common sense that he brings to this book. He has encouraged thousands in his career to look more honestly at the costs and causes of their addictions, and to be flexible in finding ways that work for each of them as they try to make better lives.

In closing, for those who are looking for real help as they strive to heal their addictions, this book is a Gift. But decide for yourself. Read the first page and see if it offers you something that matters. And if it does, read the next page—and Godspeed on your journey to recovery.

Edward Teyber, Ph.D., is an author and a clinical psychologist. He is also a professor of psychology and the director of the Community Counseling Center at California State University, San Bernardino.

INTRODUCTION

What you do in this life matters.
—Robert Downey, Jr. in *Charlie Bartlett*

I was busy running a growing company. I rarely found the time to write—or even to meditate. Then one night I felt an acute, sharp pain in my gut. It felt to me like a hole—a hole in my soul. Suddenly, it was like an awakening from a deep spiritual sleep. This revelation would inspire me to (among many other things) write again.

Before that day, I had been chasing after something intangible that I could not seem to find. But now, I could imagine, even picture, a hole in my soul—a hole I had been trying to hide, trying to fill, trying to deny.

Later, as I thought about the people I knew and the clients I had worked with over the years—especially those suffering from drug and alcohol addictions—I realized that we all have holes in our souls to some degree. Just as Herman Melville wrote in the classic *Moby-Dick,* "We are all somehow dreadfully cracked about the head, and sadly need mending."

Some of us have big holes, or "cracks," some little holes, some many holes, large and small, like Swiss cheese, and we spend our lives trying to fill these holes. Some of us are lucky. The holes are small and shallow enough to fill with friends, family, a career, hobbies, sports, exercise, religion, or faith.

Others are less fortunate. For them, the holes are too big, too many, and too deep. Nothing fills them. These people may fall in love, have a winning sports season, or even a religious revelation, and for a while live on cloud nine. The holes seem to disappear. But something always happens: the lover looks the other way, the team has a bad run, or the faith simply doesn't withstand the trials of everyday life. Then we crash, and the holes open and dominate our lives again with the pain of gaping emptiness. We may want to die. It can be *that* painful.

How Do the Holes in Our Soul Relate to Addiction?

Addiction is one way to fill in the holes in our soul. At first, drugs and alcohol fill the holes so completely that we don't even feel the pain anymore. But when we stop using, stop gambling, or whatever, we again feel the intense pain of the holes returning.

If we are lucky, we get counseling, treatment, or go to AA. If we're unlucky, we end up using again, in jail, prison, or the hospital.

What are these holes, or "cracks," in our soul? They are part of the natural human condition. No one can avoid them. We all have them. The only difference is how big the holes become, how many there are, and how we learn to fill them up. We can fill them up with love—or drugs and alcohol.

Where Do These Holes Come From?

When a baby cries and no one answers—this is when the first hole begins. Even if someone does answer, eventually no one is there to ease our pain and experience of aloneness. It cannot be avoided. Big holes are caused by continual neglect or emotional, physical, or sexual abuse. Multiple holes of different sizes result from inconsistent experiences of love, loss, and disappointment in the earliest years of life.

Sometimes these deficiencies are minimized by a strong hereditary constitution, or a strong loving family. One may have only a few, without any traumatic experiences early in life. But few people are so lucky.

How Can We Fill the Holes in Our Soul in Healthier Ways?

In the past, we turned to alcohol, drugs, sex, food, gambling, shopping, the Internet, or other forms of addiction and self-medication to fill these holes. We often got stuck in one place, repeating the same self-defeating mistakes. The way to recovery is to take a look at each of the key areas of our lives and try to identify where we are stuck—and to begin a process of change—no matter how small the steps we begin to take. Change is difficult—and scary. It may require letting go of things or people or beliefs that have given us false comfort or security. Change may require starting over again. It is not easy.

There are many positive things we can do to begin this process. We can enter addiction treatment and take sobriety seriously. We can get professional help from a psychologist, social worker, counselor, or psychiatrist. We can go to Alcoholics Anonymous (AA), Narcotics Anonymous (NA), or other anonymous fellowships or self-help meetings every day. We can get a sponsor, and let the sponsor be helpful. We can replace some of our harmful addictions with healthier behaviors such as exercising, joining a club, going to religious services, or finding creative outlets. We can read, pray, and meditate. While reading this meditation book we may discover other healthy ways to fill the holes in our soul.

What Is *Living in Balance*?

Living in Balance: 90 Meditations for Recovery from Addiction is a supplement to a larger curriculum called *Living in Balance: Moving from a Life of Addiction to a Life of Recovery* that I wrote with co-authors Mim Landry and Barry Caudill and the assistance of many others. The philosophy of *Living in Balance* is that life is never perfect—and we can only strive to find a balance among the emotional, physical, social, and spiritual aspects of ourselves. If we are having trouble in any one of these areas, we suffer and are not able to be whole. If we turn to addiction to escape our pain or discomfort, one or all of these areas is thrown out of balance.

This book is titled *Living in Balance: 90 Meditations for Recovery from Addiction* because most addictions take at least ninety days or three months of treatment and abstinence before recovery begins to take hold. Newcomers to AA or NA, especially those who come in straight off the streets without prior treatment, are often recommended to attend "ninety meetings in ninety days." This phrase is often repeated, and you're likely to hear it at a fellowship meeting. Ninety meetings and ninety meditations in ninety days is a useful guide, but ninety days is only a number. For many, it will take longer.

WHY MEDITATION?

On this journey of recovery, counselors, guides, professionals, and even friends are indispensable. Meditation and this book of reflections and affirmations can also be helpful on this journey. Abundant research shows "mindfulness meditation" or "progressive relaxation" to be effective in helping people relax, focus, and achieve balance in mind, body, and spirit to prevent relapse in recovery.

There are many types of meditation. Meditation is used for various reasons: from simple relaxation to seeking higher spiritual consciousness. Mindful meditation, Transcendental Meditation, chanting mantras, walking meditation, and other forms of religious prayer or spiritual meditation have been used for centuries. *Living in Balance: 90 Meditations for Recovery from Addiction* offers a simple meditation technique to help you prepare for recovery and provide you with practical insights to help you make important changes in your life.

HOW CAN I MEDITATE?

The meditation technique integrated in *Living in Balance: 90 Meditations for Recovery from Addiction* can be done by anyone, anywhere, and at any time. It is recommended that you frequently review the first three meditations of the book until you are meditating confidently and regularly in your daily life. All you have to do is breathe in and exhale slowly. Focus on your breathing. Take a few deep, slow breaths to get focused, but then just breathe naturally. If you are a shallow breather, or if you feel anxious, it may help to focus on your diaphragm (your belly) as it expands and contracts with your slow, deep breathing.

For a few minutes each day, focus and be entirely conscious of breathing in and breathing out. If you can, increase the number of times you meditate each day. Try meditating at your desk, before or after lunch, and during these moments try to become completely aware of your breathing. Breathe in, and feel the goodness increase in your life; then *slowly* breathe out, letting go of negative things. Breathe in your Higher Power, and *slowly* breathe out ego. Breathe in abundance, and *slowly* breathe out worries and fears. Breathe in the stars, and *slowly* breathe out anxiety and worry. Breathe in love, and *slowly* breathe out hate. It's *that* simple.

Now, make yourself comfortable, firmly place your feet on the floor, lay your hands on your lap or knees, and attend to your breathing. At this very moment, your life will begin to change. You will feel more balanced, more accepting of yourself, and more accepting of the holes in your soul and all of your beautiful imperfections.

Don't think too much about it. Just do it.

DAYS 1–30

Thought for Day 1

Make meditation a way of life and you will live more happily.

People often think meditation requires painful discipline and continuous practice. That may be partially true for more advanced levels of meditation. But meditation is also a simple practice easily integrated into your everyday life. It is more of an attitude or approach to life. Whatever you are doing, wherever you are, you only have to pause, be still, and focus on your breathing. You can even meditate with your eyes open, during a meeting, and no one will even notice. Just take a step back in your mind, focus on breathing in and exhaling as you enter a state of meditation, if only for a moment at a busy time of day. The more you do this, the more happiness you will feel. When you are in this state, you are totally in the moment, aware of your surroundings. This is not an escape; this is being fully present and in sync with the rhythm of the moment.

Affirmation

I will meditate several times today by focusing on my breathing for a few minutes. I will be aware and present in that moment.

Thought for Day 2

Through daily meditation, you expand the love in your life and reduce negative and harmful forces.

When you focus on your breathing, surrender yourself totally to the moment at hand. Daily meditation through simple breathing exercises can help you increase the positive forces in your life and reduce the negative ones. Name what you want to increase and what you want to decrease. Repeat the words. If you want to increase love in your life and decrease hate, say "love" as you breathe in and say "hate" as you exhale. Slowly repeat the word to whatever you want increased as you inhale and feel the goodness enter your soul. Exhale the negative forces, toxins, or poisons in your life. Feel them leave as you breathe out. Visualize light coming in and darkness going out. For the first few breaths, breathe in deeply and hold it for a moment. Be still. Then exhale slowly, completely, until nothing is left and hold it for another moment. Repeat this exercise a few times. Then breathe normally.

Affirmation

When I meditate, I will breathe in the good things I want in my life and breathe out the bad things that I want to eliminate.

Reflect before you react.

The power that you gain through meditation does not come only from relaxation. The more you meditate, the more you tap into an energy source that goes beyond the self. It is life energy. It may be your Higher Power, God, the collective unconscious, or nature. It is your spiritual connection. People call this energy many things—and it is difficult to describe—but through meditation you begin to feel it. This gives you strength, confidence, peace, and inner power. If everyone meditated every day, we would have much more peace in the world. Learning to meditate is a gradual process and will take time. As you practice and let yourself go, you will begin to connect to something greater than yourself. Through meditation you begin to reflect on decisions and choices that you must make in your life. Reflect on the changes you need to make—little ones and big ones. Learn to reflect before you react to events in your life.

AFFIRMATION
I will reflect on my life and actions.

Thought for Day 4

One of the most difficult things in life is to be still.

In our society, everything moves so fast. Even commercials on TV speed past us in seconds. With a million things to do, we are always on the go. We are bombarded by so much information, data, choices, decisions, and responsibilities. In our consumer society, we buy, buy, and buy. We are overwhelmed by the news, with frequent updates on the latest disasters, violence, killings, corruption, earthquakes, and more from every corner of the world. With so much constant stimulation around us, learning to relax and be still may be difficult. It is not easy to tell the world to stop and wait while we catch our breath. We have to make a real effort to be still. It requires a commitment to sit, be still, breathe in and breathe out for just a few minutes, a few times a day.

Affirmation

I will practice being still.

Living your life in balance begins with setting goals for yourself.

What do you want to accomplish in life? In what areas do you need to make changes? These questions may feel overwhelming if addiction has caused your life to collapse around you. But remember: take one step at a time. Living in balance is not about trying to be perfect. It's about progress not perfection. Set one or two goals for yourself. Do an assessment of the major areas of your life: physical, emotional, social, and spiritual. What are the most critical areas you need to improve in your physical life now: exercise, diet, sleep, smoking, drinking? What are your most pressing emotional concerns: anxiety, depression, anger, obsessions, fear? What do you want to focus on socially: intimate relationships, family relationships, work problems, conflict, or isolation? What spiritual concerns do you have: emptiness, confusion, feeling disconnected, lack of meaning, hopelessness? You may feel that you don't know where to begin. Don't worry. It will come to you.

AFFIRMATION

I will reflect on my life and identify one thing I want to change for today.

Thought for Day 6

Visualization without action is only fantasy.

Don't try to change too many things in your life at once. Think about what is most important to you right now. Set only one or two goals. Make them small and realistic—something that you can accomplish. Start with baby steps if necessary. Write these goals down. Then reflect on them. It helps to visualize yourself accomplishing these goals. Picture yourself having met the goals. Do you like what you see? Do you like how it feels? If so, go for it. If you want to accomplish these goals, you must act to bring them about. Work toward these goals. Make a plan. Take action. Evaluate your progress. Meditation is an important part of developing a vision for your life. It can help you to focus on your vision and goals. Focus on your breathing, relax, and then visualize your goals.

Affirmation

I will write down one or two realistic goals that I want to accomplish in the next ninety days.

Thought for Day 7

Sometimes, in overcoming an addiction, it helps to replace it with a healthier alternative.

If you are trying to make changes in your life, sometimes it helps to substitute a harmful behavior with a healthier one. If you are addicted to nicotine, alcohol, or another drug, it may be extremely difficult to just quit and stay quit. Even if you are successful in overcoming the withdrawal and are able to cleanse your body of the drug, ongoing cravings can sometimes overwhelm you. It's wise to replace that addiction with something healthier. For some people, it's necessary to take medication to avoid going back to a more harmful drug. The medication may be as simple as a nicotine patch or gum. Sometimes regular physical exercise, such as walking or running, can help. You may find fellowship with peers or religious and spiritual practices beneficial. A new hobby or class may help. There is no simple solution or formula. Meditation can help you find the right solution for you.

Affirmation

I will find a healthier and more meaningful alternative to my unhealthy addiction.

Thought for Day 8

Making so many decisions can be overwhelming.

How many decisions does a person make in one day? Ten? One hundred? One thousand? We make at least hundreds of small decisions every day. We often make several important decisions every day too. From time to time, life-changing decisions come along. Should I act or not? Should I go this way or that way? Should I ask him? Should I tell her? Some decisions are very difficult. Some may have serious consequences. Meditation can help you make small and big decisions. It will not magically give you answers, but it will help you to think more clearly about your decisions. Meditate throughout the day, a few minutes here, and a few minutes there. For important decisions, it is often best to apply the "twenty-four-hour rule." Sleep on important decisions, and wait twenty-four hours before making them final. If you are overwhelmed with too many decisions to make, just focus on one at a time. The rest can wait.

Affirmation

I will strive to make more thoughtful decisions in my life.

You may never fully know the impact of some decisions you make—or don't make.

When you have a tough decision to make, focus carefully on its impact on others. Think about the pros and cons, the potential consequences. Who will be affected and how? Can you predict what the long-term implications will be? Some of us worry too much about what others will think about the decisions we make. Then, we make decisions based on what others think instead of what we think is best. Sometimes it is helpful to get advice from others you trust, but only you can know what is truly best for yourself and the people you care most about. Meditate. Ask your Higher Power for guidance. Once you make your decision—for better or for worse—meditation will help you accept it and live with the decision and its consequences.

AFFIRMATION

Today I will think about an important decision I'll make in my life and the potential consequences for myself and others.

Thought for Day 10

One of the most difficult things to accept is that life never happens exactly the way we would like it to.

Throughout life we must make many compromises. The expression "you can't have your cake and eat it too" is true in many ways. Whether it is in our relationships, families, or jobs, we always have to make compromises. Even within ourselves, we have to accept our imperfections, and even our own contradictions. Sometimes we have to make choices between different options when neither choice is ideal. The way to happiness and peace is to accept that our lives, our world, will never be perfect. We must always strive to make things better, but we must also be realistic about our limits. When we become aware of a hole in our soul, it is often frightening at first. "How will I ever fill this hole?" we ask ourselves. Integrating meditation into your daily life and routine will help you to become more aware and accepting of life's limitations. It will also give you energy to take on life's challenges.

Affirmation

Today I will meditate on one compromise that I could make that will help me to live more in balance with myself and others.

Thought for Day 11

Convictions define us—yet compromises allow us to live with others and ourselves.

A favorite prayer in addiction recovery is the Serenity Prayer—"God, grant me the serenity to accept the things I cannot change, courage to change the things I can, and wisdom to know the difference." There are some things in life that we must fight for no matter what the obstacles: justice, freedom, respect, and love. There are some things where we draw the line and cannot compromise our values and beliefs. This does not mean we have to impose those values and beliefs on others, but we have to stand by our own convictions. At the same time, we must also recognize when it is better to "accept" that we cannot have everything we want in life. We also need to recognize when to respect the rights and wishes of others. The greatest challenge is to know when to stand firm and when to accept or compromise—and finally to have the "wisdom to know the difference."

Affirmation

Today I will think about what things in my life are really important—where I cannot compromise—and what things are not so important.

Thought for Day 12

Temptation is a powerful force of energy.

How do you overcome temptation? How can you control your urges, desires, and cravings? There are no easy answers to these questions. There are no simple solutions. People have tried many types of extreme behaviors to try to control their impulses. The first thing that can help is to acknowledge these desires. Temptation and cravings are a natural part of being human and being in recovery. Many people try to deny these desires or feelings—and this type of repression can cause people to act in strange and sometimes self-destructive ways. So admitting and acknowledging them is a first step. Practicing breathing and meditation will help you see and experience temptations and desires in a more objective light so that you become more aware of them. Remember, most urges and desires are a basic part of human nature, but sometimes they can take on such a powerful force that they can be harmful to you or other people.

Affirmation

Today I will accept the reality of my desires.

I am who I am at this moment in time.

There may be many things that we don't like about ourselves. We think, I'm too this or I'm too that. I'm not enough this or not enough that. There may be things that we strongly dislike about ourselves. But we are who we are and there is nothing we can do about that fact. What has been done has been done. The path to recovery begins with total acceptance of the person we are, no matter how ugly or bad or mean or weak. We must learn to forgive ourselves. And no matter what we have done, we may need to seek and ask for forgiveness from others. We need to show compassion for others and understand that they, too, are only human. But to begin the journey, we have to face the truth about ourselves and accept the person we see in the mirror. We need to explore those feelings without judgment or condemnation.

AFFIRMATION

Today I will meditate and face the truth about the person I really am.

Thought for Day 14

The most complex problems often have simple solutions.

Sometimes we get lost in the complexity of our problems. We may need to step back and envision a more simple solution that we've been missing. Sometimes we just need to have a more open mind and realize that there may be other solutions to a problem. Meditation can help you open your mind. As you meditate, invite yourself to open your mind to new possibilities. When you meditate, put aside your problem and just focus on your breathing. Breathe in naturally, and exhale as slowly as you can. When thoughts arise, let them go. Visualize them as little bubbles popping in the air. If you are dealing with a problem, tell yourself that you want to open your mind to new solutions or ideas. Don't force a decision, but let other possibilities come to you. Realize that there are many different ways to solve a problem. Release the tension and anxiety that comes from feeling the pressure to perform or succeed.

Affirmation

I will tell myself that today I will do the best that I can, and for now that is all I will ask of myself.

Thought for Day 15

Sometimes life seems too overwhelming.

Sometimes it seems like everything has gone wrong and there is no way it could ever be turned around. We may have made mistakes, big mistakes. We may have done things we are ashamed of doing. We may feel overwhelmed by so many problems, so many bills to pay, so many things to fix. Sometimes it seems like it is not even worth trying anymore. For anyone who has struggled with addiction, who has suffered losses, or who has experienced failure, these are common feelings. It all seems so overwhelming. So how do we even begin to overcome these feelings? First, we simply start with accepting and acknowledging these feelings. We recognize and say that we feel overwhelmed. Then, we take one small problem of the larger issue and see if we can do something about the smaller piece, even if it is only to make it a little better. We just take on one small problem at a time.

Affirmation

I accept that I feel overwhelmed at times and will work on one small problem today.

Thought for Day 16

The emotion of guilt can feel overwhelming at times.

Anyone who is in recovery from addiction suffers from feelings of guilt. This is because we have inevitably done many things that we regret. In early recovery, these things may even seem unforgivable. Sometimes it is necessary to forgive yourself for not only the things you have done, but also for things that you have not done and wish you did, such as visiting or saying something to a parent before he or she died. Guilt often serves an important purpose; sometimes it can serve as a warning not to do something harmful to ourselves or someone else. But guilt can also be counterproductive when it becomes overwhelming and makes you feel miserable. Understand that we are not perfect and that we all have our weaknesses and failings. We have all done things that we regret. Humans are complex beings. We do many things that we don't understand. Begin the process of forgiveness through your meditation. Seek forgiveness from yourself, from your Higher Power, and from others.

Affirmation

Today I will identify one thing that I feel guilty about and forgive myself.

Thought for Day 17

Real forgiveness comes through love.

When you begin to seek forgiveness from others or from your Higher Power, your feelings of guilt will begin to dissolve and eventually be replaced with love. To make changes in your life, you may need to begin through a process of forgiveness. Focus on forgiveness in your meditation. This will take time. So just take it one day at a time. You will begin to free yourself from destructive guilt and replace it with positive energy and love. Be sensitive to the timing of asking someone for forgiveness. If this person is still angry with you, he or she may not be ready or able to listen to you. It may help to have someone mediate between the two of you. And sometimes, you may have to accept that the other person will not forgive you until he or she believes you have made real changes in your life.

Affirmation

Today I will ask someone for forgiveness for something I have done to him or her in the past.

Thought for Day 18

I am exactly where I need to be at this very moment in time.

We may wish that we could change the past, and we often wish that we could predict or control the future, but we can't. We have to let go of past regrets and not worry so much about the future. All we really have for sure is this moment. In this moment everything is exactly as it is: good, bad, beautiful, ugly, happy, sad, warm, cold, friendly, mean, peaceful, violent, full of life or death. Whatever the reality is at this moment, this is reality. This is where I am and where I need to be at this moment in time. The more we can accept our present moment and reality and not try to fight it, judge it, or deny it, the more at peace we will be with ourselves and the world. We are safe in the here and now. Breathe in acceptance of the moment, and breathe out the past regrets and future fears. Breathe in your Higher Power, and breathe out ego.

Affirmation

I accept the total reality of my life at this very moment.

The hardest thing about moving forward is letting go of the past.

Grief is a natural response to loss. When we lose someone due to death, separation, breaking up, or even moving away, we may feel painful grief. Sometimes this grief may seem to never go away, but generally, over time, grief and pain will naturally lessen and subside. When it does not go away over the natural course of time, this may be due to unresolved grief or other issues. This can occur when the loss is very traumatic, such as an automobile accident or a violent death, or if there were unresolved conflicts in the relationship when it ended. You may feel that you never had the opportunity to do or say the things you really wanted to while you were together. Losing a parent or loved one during critical times growing up can have lifelong consequences. These experiences can widen and deepen the holes in our soul. Unresolved grief may require extra professional help and may take more time.

AFFIRMATION

Today I will reflect on the losses in my life that are keeping me from moving forward with my life.

Thought for Day 20

Death is the greatest loss in life.

It has been said that God or nature allows us to age gracefully, leading eventually to a near infant state, as we gradually lose our memory and strength, so that it will be easier to accept death. Death becomes a natural next step. When you lose someone to death in old age, it is easier to accept. But if you have lost someone in your life before he or she was ready to go—or before you were ready to let this person go—the experience can be more painful. This grief can create a hole in your soul. If the person died young or unexpectedly, it can be overwhelming. It may be nearly impossible to imagine your life without this person in it. It can be so traumatic that it may take a very long time, even many years, to overcome this trauma. In the past, you may have turned to alcohol or drugs, gambling or sex, to deal with this grief, but you know now that these addictive behaviors don't make grief go away—and can sometimes make it much worse. Don't be afraid to ask for help now. It may make all the difference in your life.

Affirmation

Today, while meditating, I will visualize the person I have loved and lost—and will feel my love for him or her.

Thought for Day 21

We all make mistakes—some big ones and many little ones.

All of us make mistakes every single day. The key to dealing with mistakes is not to try to avoid them, but to learn from them. If you mess up and fall down, get back up. See how you can learn and grow from the mistakes you make. Every problem eventually has a solution. If you are lucky, you may be able to turn a mistake into an opportunity for growth. If you can be honest with yourself and others and acknowledge your mistake, you may be surprised how people will respond to you. People are often willing to give you another chance—sometimes many chances—if you are sincere in your apology and willingness to do things differently in the future. If you can accept your own mistakes and aren't afraid to make other mistakes, you can learn from these experiences and make better decisions in the future.

Affirmation

Today I will accept my mistakes—and look for an opportunity to learn from them.

Thought for Day 22

Some mistakes simply cannot be corrected.

Sometimes mistakes may result in permanent damage to yourself or another person. The damage may not be repairable. One mistake can sometimes fracture a relationship irreparably—beyond amends-making. "There may be some wrongs you can never fully right," says the Big Book of Alcoholics Anonymous. Has this happened to you in your drinking or drug-using days? Now, you may not be able to ask for or receive forgiveness—and that may be difficult to accept. But you can still learn from the mistake. Your daily meditation will help you to more calmly face even the most terrible mistakes from your past. You can still try to improve yourself and your life by acknowledging the behavior that led to the mistake and seeing how you can live differently now without drinking or using drugs so that you are not as likely to keep on making similar mistakes. It is amazing what challenges in life people are able to overcome. The human capacity for both error and repair is vast. Accepting your humanness can help you to embrace your real and imperfect self.

Affirmation

Today I will reflect on one mistake in my life that seems beyond repair—and commit myself not to make that same mistake again.

Hope is the belief that things will work out for the better.

Having hope in the future sometimes requires blind faith and trust. Everyone has moments when all hope seems lost, but it is still better to live in hope than to live in fear. We may have dark days or moments when it is impossible to imagine things working out in a positive way. Many people turn to their faith in their God for hope. Some find hope by believing that God has a reason for everything that happens. Some look to the beauty of nature and creation for hope. Perhaps you can find hope within yourself, with a sponsor, or in your Twelve Step meeting. Realize that you are doing the best you can—trying to learn and live in a new recovery. Wherever you find hope, let it grow. Like fanning a fire, let it take over and warm your life and soul. When you meditate, focus on inhaling the good things in life and exhaling the bad, and hope will begin to emerge naturally.

AFFIRMATION

Today I will look for signs of hope in my life—and let them gain energy and grow.

Thought for Day 24

The difference between living well and just *living is good health.*

When we are young, we rarely think about the importance of good health unless we have an accident or a rare disease. But as we age we begin to realize just how important it is to have good physical health. It can mean the difference between enjoying life and hating life. Suffering from pain, illness, weakness, or disease can cast a shadow over your life that can be difficult to overcome. That is why it is so important to take care of your body now that you're in recovery. Eat well, sleep well, exercise, don't smoke, take medications as prescribed, and see your doctor and dentist regularly. We often don't recognize how important these things are until we start to feel their lack in our lives, and then it is sometimes too late. We have to do everything we can to take care of our physical bodies. We have to respect our bodies as they carry us through life.

Affirmation

Today I will do something that is good for my physical health.

Sleep is one of the most precious gifts in our lives.

Sleep restores our body and soul. If we lack sleep, we cannot function nearly as well. Lack of sound sleep is associated with many physical and emotional problems, including addiction. For most of us, a good night's sleep is, on average, seven to eight hours. Some people need more or less sleep, but it is critical to know how much your body needs to restore itself. Be sure to get the sleep that you need. Sleep allows you to dream, which is one important way that your soul works through the challenges in your life and cleanses your mind. People in early recovery often suffer from insomnia. They may not be used to falling asleep without drinking themselves into oblivion. They either can't fall asleep or they wake up too early or continually throughout the night. If you suffer from insomnia, try to reduce the things in your life that cause too much mental stimulation and stress before bedtime, such as too much TV, time on the computer, or arguments. Try meditating an hour before you're ready for bed.

AFFIRMATION

Today I will identify one thing to change in my life so that I can get the hours of sleep that I need for my body and soul.

Thought for Day 26

Emotions can be hard to control, and even harder to understand.

Emotional balance is a difficult thing to maintain, especially when you are confronted with crises or challenges in life, such as a substance use disorder and/or a mental health disorder. If we react emotionally to events in extreme ways, we can become helpless victims. If we try to deny or control our emotions too much, we can become bullies or become insensitive. Sometimes it takes great strength to absorb intense events in life, and to allow ourselves to experience the full emotional impact without becoming overwhelmed. Sometimes we need to lean on people or even take medication to get through traumatic experiences. That's okay. We may need extra time to regain our balance. When we do find our balance, we generally feel better about ourselves and are better able to accomplish personal goals. Emotional balance can be a struggle at times—and easy at other times. Try to be aware of what triggers your emotions, what influences them, and how to find the right balance for yourself.

Affirmation

I will allow myself to experience my emotions today without feeling overwhelmed. During my meditation, when an emotion arises, I will let it be.

Thought for Day 27

Many of our reactions to other people arise from our unconscious self.

When we have strong emotional reactions to other people, such as love, hate, anger, jealousy, attraction, and even "chemistry," we may be experiencing deep unconscious emotions based on episodes from childhood. These are real feelings, triggered by real people in our lives, but our emotional reactions are often influenced or colored by our earlier experiences. When we feel neglected, abandoned, abused, or even loved, nurtured, and cared for, we are often reliving these feelings as they were experienced when we were younger and more vulnerable. We may be seeking to heal painful wounds from childhood through relationships later in life. This is not a bad or unusual thing. However, in early recovery, in the first ninety days, emotional turbulence and unmanageability can often leave us vulnerable to relapse. Call your sponsor and attend a meeting when you feel emotionally vulnerable. Attend a meeting every day until you've regained some stability and strength. Gaining an awareness of how these early experiences influence our relationships later in life can help us stay sober, to grow, learn, and relate to others in deeper and more satisfying ways.

Affirmation

I will become more aware and accepting of my emotional reactions to the people in my life.

Thought for Day 28

Sometimes the simplest actions can make a big difference to another person.

We often underestimate the impact of a kind word or gesture on another person. Even those we love most—our partner, child, parent, or friend—can be taken for granted, and we miss opportunities to help them feel good. "Thank you" or "I'm sorry" or "You look nice today" and "I love your smile" are simple words that can have a big impact on a person's mood. "I missed you today" or "I love you" or "You bring joy to my life" can help a loved one feel appreciated. A touch on the shoulder, a wink, or a hug can make all the difference in a person's day. Try it. It sounds simple enough. In early recovery, we have to be careful not to become indifferent, insensitive, thoughtless, or absorbed in our own world of problems. It is too easy to get caught up in the stress and endless details of the first ninety days of recovery that we don't even notice the positive things around us—and the people we care about. Don't forget or neglect these simple actions that can make all the difference to the people we love.

Affirmation

I will make an extra effort to show at least one little sign of affection to someone I love and care about—someone I haven't acknowledged lately.

Sometimes little steps are not enough, and we have to make big changes in our lives.

In early recovery, taking small steps, even tiny steps, is critical when making changes in our lives. You may have heard others say not to make big changes in the first year of recovery because change can be too stressful and leave you vulnerable to relapse. However, at other times we must take a big dramatic step. Occasionally, we need to relocate where we live, change jobs, or end negative or destructive relationships with drinking or drug-using friends. In these cases, a small step isn't enough. These situations can require extremely difficult or painful decisions and actions. These actions may take strength, resources, and courage. Often they require several attempts to accomplish them. Often they mean giving up something that fulfills deep needs that we have and we are afraid to live without. Often we need encouragement from friends and family, help from our sponsors and fellowship, and emotional support to make these changes. But time does heal, meditation can help, and sometimes we have to let go to move forward in our own growth.

AFFIRMATION

I will meditate and reflect on my life situation to assess whether I need to make any major changes in my recovery for my own personal growth and well-being.

Thought for Day 30

To create new possibilities, first we have to be open to them.

Serendipity is the divine coincidence that makes connections in our lives and creates new possibilities. It is amazing how we cross paths with different people at critical times in our lives. A person suddenly appears in our life at just the right time. But to benefit from these relationships, first we must be open to them. When a person crosses your path, whether it is someone asking you for money on the street or a person of power inviting you into his or her world, there may be something for you to learn or gain from your encounter with this person. If you travel and fly a great deal, you may like to keep to yourself by reading, writing, or listening to music. But every now and then, take the time to get to know the person sitting next to you on the bus or plane or even standing behind you in line at the grocery store. Have some meaningful encounters with people from different walks of life. There is always something to learn from someone with life experiences different from your own. Be open to these graceful encounters. They may help keep you in your recovery in unexpected ways.

Affirmation

The next time I encounter someone whom I might ignore, I will instead seek to listen and learn something from this person.

DAYS 31–60

Happiness is when you find the right balance between love, work, and play.

Meaning in life is mainly derived from the loving relationships we have with our partners, family and friends, and Higher Power. Satisfaction in life comes mainly from feeling like we are making a contribution through our work—whether it is in a job or profession, working in the home, raising children, volunteer work, or simply working in the garden. Joy comes from being able to play and laugh and sing and dance. Meaning, satisfaction, and joy combined together bring happiness. Most of us only experience this happiness during brief periods of time in our lives—and that is natural. We would go crazy if we were happy all of the time. Oftentimes, one area of our life is out of balance, and we normally feel less happy for a period of time. But sometimes two or three of these areas are out of balance—which can lead to more intense feelings of being overwhelmed, depressed, and anxious. We may even feel as if our life is falling apart. At these times, help from a professional can get us back into balance. There is no simple formula to find this happy balance; we just do the best that we can.

AFFIRMATION

When I feel out of balance, I will love a little deeper, work a little harder, or have a little more fun.

Thought for Day 32

Service to others can give meaning in life to you and to others.

Sometimes we are simply too caught up in our own problems. We think that no one has it as bad as we do. As bad as your problems get, there are always others whose situations and suffering are worse. This is not to suggest that we minimize or ignore our own problems. Not at all. We must face them head on and deal with them as directly as we can. But it is also important that we sometimes rise above our own problems to help others less fortunate or in need of our time and attention. Keep in mind that family and friends may need us, just as much as strangers in our communities or anywhere in the world. When we were using drugs or drinking, we had little concern for others. Now, in recovery, take some time to do something for someone else, without any specific benefit for yourself. This attitude will bring you greater fulfillment in life too. Step Twelve encourages us to carry the message of recovery "in all our affairs." You don't need to wait, you can start now. Take up a cause you believe in, volunteer at a local shelter or school, or simply run an errand for someone you care about.

Affirmation

Today I will do something for someone else.

Persistence pays off.

One of the lessons we learn in life is that if you really want to accomplish something, keep trying until you can do it. If you give up too easily, you will not accomplish your goals. Some things just take practice and persistence. You have to practice over and over, again and again, until you learn to do something correctly or even perfectly. It is our natural tendency to get tired, bored, or frustrated when we don't get something right after several tries. But if we stick with it, work hard, and keep getting up every time frustration knocks us down, then we will eventually succeed. Still, be realistic. Some goals will not be accomplished. We will never be able to do or get everything we want. We may have to make tough choices about what's most important to us. But for those things you really want to do, keep trying until you get it right.

AFFIRMATION

I will renew my commitment to meditate daily and keep trying to accomplish something that I really desire.

Thought for Day 34

Believe in yourself.

One of the biggest obstacles to success is the lack of confidence in ourselves. We have all experienced failure and disappointment. Perhaps you have relapsed before and now doubt yourself. What makes some people give up and others keep going forward? Confidence, faith, love, hope—all of these things are essential. Many of the greatest accomplishments in the world were built on the experience and lessons of failure. From homeless to helpless to hopeless—the key is to believe in yourself. When you are down, reach out for any help you can find, pull yourself back up, and take the next step forward. Don't be afraid to use a cane, a walker, a wheelchair, medication, support groups, counseling, spiritual guidance—whatever you need to keep going in your recovery. If something is holding you back, say to yourself, "This is not going to keep me down." Believe in yourself, believe in your fellowship and in your Higher Power, and you will be able to accomplish unbelievable things beyond your imagination. "We will be amazed before we are half way through," states the Big Book of AA. "We are going to know a new freedom and a new happiness."

Affirmation

I believe in myself. I can do this. I know that I can.

Make a plan for your life.

If you have set goals for your life and you have faith and confidence in yourself, it may help to make a plan. Without a plan you may waste time, energy, and feel frustrated with your lack of progress. Of course you can't plan for everything. Plans have to be flexible to adapt to changing reality. But it is usually best to start out with a plan, even a simple one. Pick one or two of your major goals in life, such as getting your life in better balance physically, emotionally, socially, or spiritually. The goal may be related to your career, business, marriage, or recovery. Write down your goals as clearly as you can. Break the larger goals down into smaller objectives that will help you reach your goals. Identify the steps you need to take to meet these objectives. Write down every step. Take an inventory of your assets. Get help with the plan from someone who may have relevant experience, possibly someone else in recovery. It usually takes much longer than we would hope, but keep trying.

AFFIRMATION

Today I will identify one goal and make a plan related to achieving it for myself. And I will continue to meditate, to breathe in confidence, and to breathe out fear.

Thought for Day 36

As you begin your recovery process, think about finding a place to go that will help you succeed and feel safe and centered.

When a woman close to me decided to stop using heroin for good, after many years of addiction, she was living in Michigan. The only way she could quit successfully was to completely change her environment. She drove with me to North Carolina and spent one week at my apartment, suffering through withdrawal, until she felt well enough to drive on her own. Then she drove on to Florida, found a little apartment on the beach, and started her life over again, without drugs. It wasn't easy for her, but she did it. She got a job, got married, had beautiful children, and overcame many new challenges in her life. She had tried to quit many times before. But only when she changed her life dramatically did she succeed. You may not need to drive across the country, but it is essential that you find a safe and secure place to succeed in your recovery.

Affirmation

Today I will meditate on what I need to change in my life to maintain my recovery from addiction.

Character is the part of us that keeps our commitments.

We make many commitments in life. Some commitments are easy to keep. Some can be very hard. Sometimes we make a commitment to something or someone at a time in our lives when that commitment makes total sense. Then circumstances change. People change. You may reach a point after many years where the commitment you once made no longer makes sense. Do you just turn your back on the commitment? Do you walk away from it? These questions can be heart-wrenching and lead to tough decisions. It's the character in us that helps us to honor our commitments. Without such character, no one could rely on us for anything. No one would know who we are or what we stand for. But when the commitment no longer makes sense or comes into conflict with other critical values or choices, you must face this conflict with honesty, integrity, and oftentimes with support and guidance.

AFFIRMATION

Today, when I meditate, I will feel the strength of my character fill my soul—and let it guide me to face the commitments I have made in my life.

Thought for Day 38

Every breath of life gives us energy.

One of the things in life that we most naturally take for granted is breathing. How precious is each breath? If you have ever been on the brink of death, you already know the answer. Each breath gives us life-sustaining energy. We all know the expression, "Take time to smell the roses." Well it is also important to take time to breathe. Notice the life force of your breathing. Close your eyes and focus on your breathing now. Take in a normal breath, and slowly release the air from your body. Very slowly. Don't tense up; take your time. When you breathe in, feel the strength it gives you—feel the energy. What a gift it is to have this breath—this life energy. Take several breaths, and release each one slowly. Just enjoy the moment of peace that this can bring to your day. This is the simplest form of meditation. Do this a few times a day, and you will notice that it gives you more energy. Just like when you eat something delicious and chew it slowly to get the full flavor and pleasure of the food—enjoy the gift of your breathing and the energy it brings.

Affirmation

Today I will take the time to appreciate the gift of breathing.

Observe your reactions to people, places, and things.

One of the most challenging parts of recovery from addiction is dealing with the people, places, and things that can spark your desire and craving to smoke, use drugs, or drink alcohol. Do you know that research shows the pleasures of your addiction become associated with and are triggered by certain people, places, or things? During the early stages of recovery, it is generally best to avoid these people, places, and things that make you want to go back to your addiction. This may be difficult if they are a major part of your life, but it may also be necessary. If you can't avoid them, then you will have to learn how to manage your urges and desires when they are triggered. Aside from calling your sponsor, using distraction, and saying the Serenity Prayer, meditation is a good first step for learning to control your urges to use. It will take much practice, but you may learn to counter your urges through meditation at least temporarily until the urge passes or at least reduces to a manageable level. Always be aware of the people, places, and things that trigger your addiction. It helps to write them down.

AFFIRMATION

Today I will be more aware of the people, places, and things that trigger my thoughts and desire to go back to my addiction.

Thought for Day 40

People tend to deny or run away from pain, but accepting that pain is inevitable and will help to ease it away.

It's no surprise that we will do almost anything to avoid both physical and emotional pain. We will take medicines, prescribed or not, to make the pain go away. We will escape by jumping from one relationship to another, one job to another, one place to another. It seems too hard to sit and feel the pain. It can be too hard to deal with the pain that can come up in relationships. It is especially hard to admit the pain that we cause ourselves and others. It is much easier to reach for a drink or drug, open the refridgerator, or find other distractions. But when we take the time to feel the pain, to understand and acknowledge the pain, it is more likely to dissipate and ease up over time. If you can sit still with your pain, talk about it, and accept it, the pain will soften.

Affirmation

If I'm hurting, I will try to sit still, meditate, and let the pain soften and dissipate.

Thought for Day 41

Loneliness is an intolerable state for some people.

The ability to be alone, to enjoy ourselves, is an important attribute. People sometimes say, "I am alone, but not lonely," meaning they enjoy being with themselves. The capacity to accept one's aloneness, and even to enjoy it, is important in recovery. Some people, especially introverts, thrive on it and can be productive and energized in solitude. But some people, particularly extroverts, have a harder time being alone and feel more energized around others. Often, in addiction, loneliness creeps in and casts a dark shadow over a person. These feelings of loneliness can be very unpleasant and even painful. Many addicts drink, drug, eat, or have compulsive sex to escape feeling lonely. In early recovery, the fear of loneliness can lead to relapse. Meditation can be very helpful when you are having trouble being alone. Focus on your breathing and embrace your aloneness. Feel deeply your connection to nature or the universe.

Affirmation

Today I will be alone, in solitude, for an hour—and if I feel lonely, I will acknowledge and accept these feelings as being normal.

Thought for Day 42

How do we find the strength to carry on?

Sometimes, it may seem as if life is just not worth living. Tragic loss of someone we love, illness, chronic pain, constant stress, money problems, and addiction can wear us out. Some people just get tired of living and want to give up. Sometimes these feelings can cause a person to want to take his or her own life—to commit suicide. Sometimes a person tries to escape by relapsing into addiction. What gives those of us who feel so tired or desperate the ability to keep going? Sometimes it takes the help of someone else who cares or loves you. It can be lifesaving to accept this person's support and love. Sometimes it takes a professional counselor, sponsor, or spiritual guide to help you reach deep inside to find your core of strength and hope. Sometimes it takes reaching up to the heavens to find your Higher Power. If you feel desperate, accept this feeling as you meditate, then reach outside for help, while you reach deep inside for strength and hope.

Affirmation

Today I will take time to meditate and focus on the strength and hope deep inside myself.

How do we make the hardest choices in life?

Choices are rarely simple. They are rarely between a good choice and a bad one. The tough choices are always complicated, such as weighing this good and bad against the other good and bad. Which choice weighs more heavily on the good and tips the scale? Have you really thought about how bad the bad can get? How much pain may you cause by making one choice and not the other? How much pain might you cause by making the wrong choice? How do you know the best choice when you can't predict the future? In the throes of addiction and early recovery, you may not be able to make clear choices, or evaluate them and their consequences realistically. Critical life choices require a clear head and stable emotions. If you are early in recovery, you may need to evaluate these choices with the help of others. Where do you find your guidance, support, help, and strength? Meditation will not give you all the answers, but it can help you to be more honest and recognize the truth.

AFFIRMATION

I commit to doing whatever is necessary to clear my mind and meditate on and discuss with others the important choices in my life.

Thought for Day 44

If I am obsessed, I am likely vulnerable to relapse.

You may wonder if you are still addicted. You may have even stopped doing what you were doing—drinking, drugging, smoking, gambling, eating compulsively, or having sex compulsively. So you may think that you have overcome your addiction on your own—but it's not likely. It generally takes months or even years for a person's brain to return to a relatively normal, pre-addiction level of functioning. When you feel you are obsessing, craving, desiring, longing—then it is likely that these are signs that your brain is still craving momentary pleasure and relief. This is compounded by the ever-present holes in your soul. So what can you do? Meditate. Talk about it. Substitute something for your addiction—if it is more positive and less destructive. Take medication—if a doctor believes you need it. Whatever it takes—do it! Take care of yourself and get the help you need to get to Step One. Your path may not be a straight one to get there—but keep moving forward. Pick yourself back up—and move on. You can do it.

Affirmation

Today I will take an honest look at myself and my addictions.

Thought for Day 45

A good job is one of the most rewarding things in life. To lose this job can be devastating.

When the 2010 Gulf Coast oil spill destroyed fishing and tourist areas around the Gulf, thousands of people lost their jobs and livelihoods. "I don't know how I'm going to live," one shrimper said. A person's job or career means so much. It is our identity, how we see ourselves, our livelihood. So when a person loses a job, or can't find one because of a lack of training, lack of employment opportunities, or a criminal record, it can be devastating and depressing. How does one overcome such overwhelming challenges? There are no simple answers. Don't be afraid to explore new possibilities or industries. You may have lost a high-level management or professional job due to your addiction and now need to start over at an entry-level position. Then study, learn, practice, meditate, and network after your fellowship meetings; be as positive as possible. Take it "one day at a time." Believe that for every challenge there is a solution—eventually.

Affirmation

I will focus on my work and take one small step to make myself better, stronger, and happier.

Thought for Day 46

There are many ways to soothe pain.

During our active addiction, we soothed our pain with alcohol, drugs, or other substances. The addiction actually causes the brain to produce chemicals that relieve pain, both physical and emotional. Eventually addiction takes control over a person's life and causes him or her to make bad choices just to sustain the addiction. We became so obsessed with the need to kill the pain or to feel good, even "normal," that we forgot about other important things in life. Our lives got out of balance, and we began doing destructive things to ourselves and others. Through the support of others, fellowship, counseling, faith, love, physical rehabilitation, meditation, and dedication—you can regain your life. You can begin to get your life back into balance—physically, socially, emotionally, and spiritually. Take one step at a time, one problem at a time. Find healthier ways to tolerate pain and discomfort; find healthier ways to feel good and okay with yourself.

Affirmation

I will find new, healthier ways to soothe my personal pain.

Physical balance takes practice.

Just like learning a sport, developing physical balance in your life takes lots of practice. Even something as simple as walking takes practice. When you start out, especially if you are out of shape or haven't exercised in a long time, walking around the block can be a challenge. But if you walk slowly at first and you walk every day, it will get easier with practice. Soon you will walk faster and for longer periods of time. Then you can walk two blocks, three blocks, a mile, three miles, and even more. But "easy does it." You will become stronger and healthier over time if you just stick with it. If you have physical problems, see a doctor and get treatment. Some people have physical limitations—but there is almost always something that you can do. With practice you will get better at it. Take on one thing at a time, and "one day at a time." Practice, and you will gain confidence, and soon you will feel the difference.

Affirmation

Today, I will begin one new physical activity, and tomorrow I will practice it.

Thought for Day 48

Emotional balance requires introspection—looking inside yourself.

When we are out of emotional balance, we are generally moving too fast or too slow, or we are too high or too low. We need to be able to stop for a moment to see where we stand. We may need to look inside of ourselves to understand what is happening and how we are feeling. That's why taking an inventory of ourselves helps people in recovery. If you feel out of balance, take an inventory—take a close look at how you are feeling and what you are doing. Get in touch with your deeper feelings. Meditation may help you to be less defensive and experience your true feelings more deeply. Sometimes it may be too difficult to look at yourself and how you are feeling without the help of a counselor, sponsor, spouse, or friend. Acknowledge these feelings no matter how bad they may seem. Once you begin to look at yourself honestly, you can set goals for how to achieve better emotional balance in your life.

Affirmation

Today I will meditate on how I am feeling emotionally.

One big challenge in relationships is finding the balance between dependence and independence.

As human beings, we start out in life with a very long stage of dependency on other people, primarily our mother and father. For the first two years we are dependent on them for almost everything. We are at the mercy of others for food, drink, clothes, shelter, warmth, and love. It can be a year or two before we can even stand on our own two feet. That is a very long time. During that time, we get used to being taken care of by others. We pretend we don't like it too much—and yell "no" or "I can do it myself" or sometimes even "I hate you" when things don't go our way. As we grow older, we value our ability to do things on our own and to stand on our own two feet. But as adults, it is often difficult to find the right balance between letting ourselves be taken care of, supported, and helped—and doing things on our own. Likewise, it is often difficult to know how supportive to be toward a person you love and still give the space he or she needs to feel independent. Finding this balance of interdependence is one of the most challenging, yet fulfilling, aspects of sober adult relationships.

AFFIRMATION

Today I will talk with my partner or a loved one about the balance of dependence and independence in our relationship.

Thought for Day 50

Jealousy can be triggered when dependence and independence are out of balance.

Jealousy is one of the most intense emotions people experience in life. It can be excruciatingly painful. We often first feel jealousy with the common experience of sibling rivalry (jealousy of a brother or sister over a parent's affections). Later, this emotion can be triggered by the simple glancing affections of our partner toward another person. It is true that passionate relationships are more prone to jealousy, and yet many prefer the jealousy inside a passionate relationship than one lacking passion. Unfortunately, despite one's good intentions, this emotion can take control of your emotions like a monster. Now without the aid of drugs or drinking to make these intense feelings go away, people in recovery often must struggle to learn new and more constructive ways to handle this emotion. One thing that can be helpful is to remember that "these feelings, too, will pass." Remember: breathe in, breathe out . . .

Affirmation

The next time I feel jealous or another intense emotion, such as anger or fear, I will step back to explore and discuss how these feelings affect my most important relationships.

Thought for Day 51

Nothing feels better in life than to feel loved.

To feel loved for who you are is one of the most wonderful feelings in life. To feel accepted for who you are—the good, the bad, and the ugly—is to experience being loved unconditionally. To know that you are loved without conditions, without debts, without reservations is to feel loved. Such love gives us meaning in life, as well as joy, confidence, security, and peace of mind. Unfortunately, feeling this unconditional love is rare and commonly short-lasting. Because we all struggle with our own needs for love and security, it is often difficult to give love in such an unconditional way. We, therefore, undermine the love we give and receive with our own insecurities. As much as we may want to give unconditional love—we get angry, lose our patience, lash out, and tear the unconditional bond. On the one hand we are human and have to accept our own nature and limitations—yet we will live a richer life if we can love with an open heart and without condition.

Affirmation

Today I will open my heart to the people I love—and let them know that I love them for who they are.

Thought for Day 52

Spiritual growth does not follow a straight path.

What is spiritual growth? It is a process of finding meaning in life or feeling connected to your God or Higher Power. Some people may experience a moment of truth, a spiritual breakthrough, or a peak experience that changes them in a deep and enduring way. But for most people, spiritual experience is a gradual process with many ups and downs, insights and setbacks, times of strength and weakness, and moments of certitude and uncertainty. In recovery from addiction, relapse is often an inevitable part of the process; spiritual growth, too, takes many turns, sometime for the worse. Sometimes it may seem that there is no growth at all. Also, as with recovery, it helps to have spiritual teachers and guides to shed light where there is darkness and to help us overcome our own limited knowledge. Deep meditation can help connect you to a higher consciousness. Reading spiritual texts, including the Big Book, can also help to enlighten you on this journey.

Affirmation

Today I will meditate on my spiritual growth and ask myself if this is an area where I need to pay more attention.

Prayer and meditation are pathways to a spiritual connection.

Whether you believe in God, a higher spiritual consciousness, universal love, or basic ethical values, taking time to pray and meditate as stated in Step Eleven helps you to gain a higher awareness and spiritual connection. Martin Buber writes about the "I-Thou" experience—feeling totally at one with God, nature, or even another person. Most of the time we live in the practical, material, and realistic day-to-day world of "I-It," instead of the "I-Thou." Just getting through the mundane and ordinary life is challenging and often uninspiring. But there are moments, timeless moments, when we may feel totally connected with this other world. Practicing prayer and meditation, as instructed in Step Eleven, does not guarantee that you will feel this connection, but if you open yourself to this other world and seek such a connection, you will be more likely to experience it. Pay attention to the positive energy all around you. It can help to prepare you for this connection. "Letting God and letting go" is an expression that simply says to open yourself up to this spiritual force. Let it enter your life.

AFFIRMATION

Today I will pray and mediate for spiritual growth and guidance.

Thought for Day 54

The process of change begins with the recognition that what you are doing may not be producing the results you really want.

There is a saying that being crazy is doing the same thing over and over again and expecting different results. We get ourselves into self-destructive patterns of behavior or relationships that keep hurting ourselves or others. We have an exceptional ability to fool ourselves into believing that things will be different if we just ignore this one little problem or just try one more time. We drank and used for years believing this. The problem is that life is generally a matter of odds: you might be able to drive home drunk one or two or even three more times, but odds are that one of those times you will get arrested or crash your car, injuring yourself or others. You may have fun getting high a few times, or even many times, but stay on this road and you will become addicted, which can lead to other consequences. You may be in an abusive relationship and think that if you only stop disappointing the other person he or she will stop abusing you, but chances are that the abuse will continue. Face reality.

Affirmation

I will face the reality of my life and evaluate the likely consequences of continuing to do what I have been doing.

Reaching rock bottom is not necessary for change, but it does make you realize that you have no other choice.

Some people recognize the need to make changes in their lives without hitting rock bottom. This is a lucky thing and may spare them and others much pain and loss. This change usually comes about through pressure, warnings, or even an intervention from others. Someone may care about you and want you to be happier, or this person may simply be tired of your destructive behavior. Sometimes hearing from others over and over again that we need to change our behavior is enough to make us want to change. Sometimes it isn't. Many people decide to quit smoking when the people they care about have bugged them so much that they eventually quit. But many other people need to experience the negative consequences of their behavior before they truly recognize the need for change. They have to feel the loss of breath, health, money, status, freedom, or worse, their loved ones. If you have a chance to change before reaching rock bottom—take it.

AFFIRMATION

Today I will meditate and imagine making the changes that I know will make life better for myself and others.

Thought for Day 56

Sometimes a hole in the soul is so deep it seems like it never ends.

We all struggle to fill the holes in our soul in any way that we can. Sometimes we can fill those holes in healthy ways through work, art, music, creating things, sports, hobbies, and even love. Sometimes we fill them in unhealthy and even dangerous ways such as addictions to drugs, alcohol, gambling, food, sex, or romance that is more fantasy than reality. When we fill the holes in unhealthy and dysfunctional ways, we may feel temporary pleasure and joy, but it is usually followed by depression and despair. We feel this most painfully when we lose the thing or the person filling this hole. We go through withdrawal—sometimes deeply painful withdrawal. It seems as if all hope is lost and the sun will never rise again. In desperation, we may relapse and go right back to the unhealthy addiction, and the cycle repeats itself once again. This pain seems never to end. But it does end. In time, we heal.

Affirmation

Today, I will find one healthy activity to fill a small hole in my soul.

There is often a thin line between real love and imaginary love.

There is no better feeling in the world than to be in love. The sense of oneness, intimacy, romance, and passion is the highest high. Sometimes, though, we question ourselves, wondering whether the experience is real love or fantasy. Are you relating to this other person as he or she truly is or as you imagine him or her to be? Do you understand and accept the person, strengths and weaknesses, beauty and warts? Or do you only see what you want to see and ignore or deny the other parts? No one can know for sure. We are all driven by unconscious forces, and no one can judge but you. You have to try to be honest with yourself and your partner as best you can. In any relationship there will be ups and downs. When the love is real, it will be able to withstand these ups and downs through honest and open communication. When it is imaginary, the ups and downs may be too great for the relationship to survive. Honest communication can help to clarify the reality from fantasy.

AFFIRMATION

I will make an honest inventory of my relationships to see if they are real or if I can make them more real through honest communication.

Thought for Day 58

Recovery is a process that takes time, patience, persistence, and pain.

There is no easy way to overcome years of an addiction. The more we try to run away from it, the longer it takes and the more damage we cause. If you really want to recover from an addiction, you have to admit to it, as in Step One, accept the pain and loss, and feel the hole in your soul. It may be unbearable to handle it all at once, which is why many people relapse. At first, it seems you may never be free from the desire or craving, but in time it becomes less powerful and less frequent. In time you can gain more control (through surrender and acceptance) over your addiction rather than having it control your life. While you are going through the process of recovery, you may feel as if you are out of sync or out of touch with the world. You may feel disconnected from your old friends, family, and co-workers—and feel lonely. Your situation may feel temporarily hopeless—and you despair. But if you hang in there, stay focused on your recovery, talk with others in the fellowship, and share, these feelings will pass. You will grow stronger in time. Just take it "one day at a time."

Affirmation

Today I will make a commitment to my recovery. I will try to find healthier and more fulfilling ways to fill the holes in my soul.

Real change is a slow process.

We wish change could happen quickly and easily, but usually it doesn't work that way. Sometimes change may appear rapid, but that is usually in hindsight after the change has been evolving for months or years below the surface of your awareness. Not only is change a slow process, there may be setbacks, and sometimes it seems we learn the same lessons over and over again. This is because we have a natural resistance to change. Our defense mechanisms take over, and we are often blind to our own traps and shortcomings. It can help to speed things up when we seek the input of others in groups or therapy. Sometimes other people can help us to see things we can't see in ourselves. Often, your sponsor or fellowship meetings can provide you lifesaving feedback. Listen to the input of others, and reflect on their feedback and suggestions. You may disagree with their observations, but if you keep an open mind, you may see things you didn't see before.

AFFIRMATION

I will seek input from others, listen, and be open to change.

Thought for Day 60

If there is something really important to you that you want, you have to work for it.

If you want to achieve something or accomplish a goal, picture it in your mind, lay out a plan, and work toward your goal one step at a time. Keep working at it every day. If you need help or guidance, ask for it. If you face obstacles, think of other solutions. If you get discouraged, find hope in prayer or meditation. If you relapse, get back up and work your recovery plan. Don't give up. Keep trying. Most people take much longer to reach their goals than they expect. You may have to change your goals as you move forward and learn new things. You may realize that some of your goals are simply not realistic. You may have to make compromises. But if you really want something, work as hard as you can. It may seem as if you will never reach your goal. But many times, just when it seems out of reach, you find that it is possible.

Affirmation

I will meditate on my goals, then make a plan, and work toward them with all my heart.

DAYS 61–90

Embrace the process.

Setting goals and working toward them can be a fun, enjoyable process. Even experiencing the frustration and pain of change and recovery can be rewarding when you embrace the process. When you do, you see the "light at the end of the tunnel." Then, sobriety becomes more like a river flowing with you into a new life. Don't fight or resist it. When you accept the process and let yourself experience it, this surrender can be fulfilling in its own way. It is part of your growth: reaching a higher spiritual level of consciousness or awareness. Let go of the anxiety or fear of change as you accept that this is a part of life. It will help you become a stronger person. Fear inhibits change; acceptance allows it to happen. Know that there will be ups and downs, and appreciate the ride. Celebrate small successes in healthy ways with the people you care about.

AFFIRMATION
I will accept and embrace the process of change.

Thought for Day 62

Breathe in love; breathe out ego.

Ego is the reflection of your self, separate from the rest of the world. It contains the driven compulsive need to be loved, needed, wanted, approved of, satisfied, filled up, admired, powerful, dominant, and in control. It is the opposite of unconditional love of others, nature, or your Higher Power. Accepting unconditional love is accepting that we are part of something much bigger than ourselves. Ego pushes us to meet our own needs without consideration of the needs of others. It allows us to exploit, harm, and disrespect others, because it only cares about the self. Ego drives addiction. It seeks only pleasure and relief from pain. Sometimes our ego may feel the need for protection when we have been hurt or disappointed. But in the end, ego only serves the self and causes the self to be limited and isolated. Love is the antidote to ego. Breathe in love; exhale ego.

Affirmation

Today I will meditate on love and open myself up to the vulnerability of letting love into my life while letting go of my ego.

When we hit bottom with our addiction, it may seem as if all hope is lost.

Sometimes it seems like everything has gone wrong. We may feel depressed. Nothing we do seems to make things better. If only, we think, we could start our lives over again. We may feel so guilty over our past drug use or drinking that we just want to end the pain. Some people may even feel suicidal when they come out of deep depression and see what a mess they have made of life. That's why it's so important to talk to others, such as recovery friends or your sponsor. During these dark days, it is important to remember: time will heal the pain and things will get better. Often the darkest hour is just before the light of dawn. It is possible to rebuild your life, make amends, and move forward. You are doing it now. Through prayer and meditation, reading recovery literature, helping others, keeping faith, and taking even the smallest positive steps to improve your life, you are changing the course of your life.

AFFIRMATION

When all hope seems lost, I will focus on the simple things in life—a flower, a sunset, a star, my breath, my heartbeat—and I will be thankful for it.

Thought for Day 64

Negative thinking can lead to negative outcomes.

Some people believe that if you just think positively, then positive things will happen in your life. Life is not that simple. There is certainly a power in positive thinking, but one must work hard at things to make them happen. You have to dedicate yourself, have discipline, learn skills, and learn from your mistakes. Luck, faith, hope, and destiny all seem to play a role. You take responsibility for your life by maintaining your recovery, going to meetings, and being a good parent, friend, or employee. At the same time, negative thinking can undermine your actions. If you approach life with negative beliefs and expectations, you are more likely to have failures and negative outcomes. This doesn't mean you should take a Pollyanna approach to life, ignoring problems or denying bad or painful experiences. Acknowledge the good and the bad, but don't let negative thoughts dominate your life and recovery.

Affirmation

When I meditate, I will become more aware of my negative thoughts and reactions and how they influence my life.

Look for people in your life who can have a positive influence on you.

My beloved grandmother passed away at the ripe age of ninety-nine. She said that over the years she worked hard to clear her mind of negative thinking. She was always full of life, humor, and unconditional love because she had developed a very positive perspective on life. Even when she could no longer live independently and had to move into a nursing home, she accepted this with grace, and all of the workers in the home came to love her dearly. She spent her early years in Eastern Europe, dirt poor while her father went ahead to America to work until he could raise enough money to send for the family. Her husband, my grandfather, was an alcoholic most of his life until he was fortunate to find AA in his later years, and as a result, she faced many challenges. When my grandmother had a heart attack in her late eighties, the doctor asked her if she wanted to have heart surgery and go on living for a few more years. Of course, she said, life was too precious to let it go that easily.

AFFIRMATION

I will reach out to someone who has been a positive influence on me and thank the person for enhancing my life.

Thought for Day 66

Finding fellowship can save your life.

When I was a child, I can remember my grandfather sitting at the kitchen table with a blank stare on his face. I didn't know it, but he was probably drunk. He was a sweet man who would never harm anyone on purpose. We all loved him very much, although we rarely heard him speak a complete sentence. He drank himself into oblivion most of his life, often disappearing for days at a time. Then one day, I don't know how, he found the fellowship of Alcoholics Anonymous. The group took him in like a lost child, and he began to rebuild his life. My grandmother embraced Al-Anon. When my grandfather died several years later in his late seventies, there was a funeral procession blocks long filled with his friends from AA, including judges whom he met while helping his friends in court, and even principals from schools where he spoke to youth about his recovery from alcoholism. Fellowship for my grandfather did, indeed, save his life.

Affirmation

Today I will attend a fellowship meeting, talk with my sponsor, or find a sponsor if I don't have one yet who can help me with my recovery.

Different perspectives and opinions can be helpful in your recovery.

A diversity of perspectives and opinions can help you see more options and make better decisions. That's why a recovery group can be so helpful. At meetings you will hear lots of ideas, practices, and things people do to prevent relapse and sustain their recovery. Sometimes you will also hear important things about yourself that you may not want to hear. That's why finding a sponsor or a mentor is critical for your recovery. If you seek feedback and input from people with the same perspectives and experiences as you, then you are likely to continue in the same direction. It is important to keep an open mind, to solicit different opinions and perspectives, as you make up your own mind about things in your life. You may be afraid to discuss some personal issues because you are worried about what others will think about you, but you will be surprised by how accepting and understanding others can be, especially if they have been there before themselves. Another person may open your mind to new ideas and solutions if you allow yourself to consider these different ideas.

AFFIRMATION

Today I will not be afraid to be open to a new perspective or advice about something bothering me from my sponsor or in a fellowship meeting.

Thought for Day 68

If you don't go after what you really want, you will never get it.

What keeps us from going after what we want? Sometimes it is fear of failure. Fear of success. Fear of conflict. Fear of change. Fear of the unknown. Sometimes it is guilt. Guilt over getting something others don't have. Maybe you feel that you don't deserve to get what you want. Maybe your addiction has been the major obstacle. Understand what it is that keeps you from moving forward so that you can make a clear and conscious choice. For example, you may choose not to finish your college degree at this time. You may have your own personal reasons, such as financial ones. But know what these reasons are so that you don't live with regret over your inaction. If you understand what is holding you back, you may decide that you don't want to be held back by these reasons any longer. You may decide to face your fears, deal with your guilt, or find other ways to fulfill your responsibilities. If you choose to try to get what you want, go for it. Take a chance.

Affirmation

I will meditate on what I really want and try to understand what may be keeping me from going after it.

Giving up an addictive substance or behavior is one of the hardest things to do.

One of the toughest addictions to overcome is smoking cigarettes. The addiction to nicotine is especially difficult because cigarettes are designed to addict people quickly. We are faced with commercial influences from the cigarette industry, which does everything possible to disguise the dangers of smoking. For so many, nothing seems to help them quit, and they fail over and over again. They try every method, technique, and medication and are still unable to quit. My mother struggled like that. She tried to quit many times, never succeeding for more than a month or two, and at sixty-eight died of lung cancer. On the other hand, there are those who think they could never quit, but then one day, maybe after many efforts, they succeed. My father smoked three packs a day, non-filtered, for fifty years from the age of twelve. Then one day, he quit, against all odds. Step One asks us to admit that we are powerless over our addiction. But before you can take Step One, you have to decide that you want to give up your addictive substance or behavior. Often, this decision must be made many times.

AFFIRMATION

Today I will meditate on my addiction and reaffirm that I really want to quit my addictive substance or behavior.

Thought for Day 70

The two most powerful words in the world are "thank you."

It is amazing how powerful these two words are when said from the heart. Some even say that these two words are the only prayer we need to say at the end of the day. So often we take people for granted. We assume people know that we appreciate what they do for us. We rarely realize how much parents give us during the course of our childhood and our lives. We rarely appreciate how much we learn from siblings, teachers, friends, sponsors, and colleagues. We like to think of ourselves as self-sufficient. But in reality, we thrive on the acknowledgement, affection, attention, support, and love from those around us. Yet how often do we return this attention and affection and say thank you? How often do we acknowledge the little things that people do for us? How often do we thank our Higher Power and others for the role they played in helping with our recovery. Yet, when we do, "thank you" often means so much to the person we thank. It feels good to be appreciated. If feels good when someone notices what we have done for them.

Affirmation

Today, at least once, I will thank someone for what he or she did for me, no matter how small or big.

Thought for Day 71

Creativity comes from the soul.

Creativity is the natural flow of new and unique ideas. Sometimes these ideas are not necessarily original; sometimes it may be that they just come together in a new way. Imagine bubbles floating in the air—each with a new idea or solution. As each bubble pops, it creates new possibilities. Don't try to censor the ideas or evaluate them, just let them flow. Use meditation to release the barriers and free the creativity inside of you. Let go completely. Don't even try to think of ideas or solutions. Just enter into a deep state of relaxation and nothingness. Then, when you come out of your meditation, you may find it easier to experience new creative ideas and solutions. The free flow of creativity can help you to release yourself from narrow or limited ideas. Creativity is a way out of the box. Open your mind. Refresh your mind. Let your creativity flow.

Affirmation

Today, while meditating, I will open my mind, heart, and soul to new creative solutions.

Thought for Day 72

Self-discipline is one of the most important, but difficult, habits to learn.

Self-discipline is something we generally learn at an early age. We are lucky if we have loving parents who nurture and teach us self-discipline. Parents can teach self-discipline in several ways. They can help us learn to delay gratification and work toward goals one step at a time. They can reward us for achieving goals. They can set limits on behavior in a loving but firm way, thereby teaching us that there are limits and boundaries that we must learn to respect. Finally, they can teach us by example, demonstrating self-discipline by working persistently toward goals, even when sacrifices are required. If we didn't have the benefit of learning from our parents through loving discipline and modeling, then we have to work harder to develop these habits in ourselves. If you have children, now is the time to pass on these gifts to them.

Affirmation

I will reflect on my self-discipline in life and make any changes that are necessary to strengthen my resolve.

When we love and feel loved, we feel whole.

Many of us search for love our whole lives. Sometimes we find it only for fleeting moments, or for months or years. When we give our love to someone completely and we feel loved by that person in return, there is no other feeling like it in the world. We feel complete, whole, vibrant, and alive. That kind of connection is what most of us seek and rarely find. Why is it so difficult to find and keep that kind of complete love? Basically people are self-centered. It is our human nature. Our egos get in the way. As addicts and alcoholics, for many years our need for drugs or alcohol took priority over our relationships. Even in recovery, when we want to give our love totally to others, our own needs still tend to take precedence and override our love of others. The Big Book calls it "self-will run riot." As we struggle to set aside our own needs to give love to partners, friends, family, and especially our children, we have to do the best we can to balance meeting our own needs with giving unconditional love to others around us.

Affirmation
Today I will give a little extra love and attention to the people whom I love.

Thought for Day 74

The first step to Step One is to look in the mirror.

What do you see when you look in the mirror? Are you happy, sad, confident, afraid, proud, or ashamed? The first step is to accept what you see and who you are no matter how terrible your past might be. We are what we are. Step One requires an honest look at ourselves, as we begin to accept and change our character defects and shortcomings. We may have done terrible things during our drinking and drugging days, and as a result, we may have unbearable feelings of shame or guilt. We may feel lost or alone. Still, we have to start with who we are. The Twelve Step fellowships and other recovery programs give people in early recovery the skills to heal, make amends, and move forward. Acceptance is the core to Step One. You are human. You are not perfect. You are not complete. You are learning. You are what you are at this moment, nothing more, nothing less. That is the starting point. Don't be afraid to embrace what you see because acceptance begins the process of change.

Affirmation

Today, I celebrate who I am, even if only for a moment.

The biggest obstacle to change is fear.

Fear keeps us stuck in our feelings, in negative patterns, and out of balance. Overcoming fear may seem like trying to fly. It goes against our nature. Fear is a self-reinforcing defense mechanism. The more we deny our fear, the stronger it takes hold of us. The more we push it away, the more it pushes back. The best way to deal with fear is to permit it to be and accept what it is—a disabling emotion. First, acknowledge your fear. Then, if you begin to feel anxious, sit down and allow yourself to experience the anxiety for a short while. We are all afraid at times. Perhaps there is a person or an approaching event that worries you. We may not admit it or even be aware of it at times, but fear is unavoidable and part of being human. The more you accept and feel your fear, the less of a grip it will have on your life. If there is something you want to do but are afraid to do, accept your fear. Listen to your fears, but don't let them control you.

AFFIRMATION

I will not run from my fears, but embrace and accept them.

Thought for Day 76

Healing from traumatic experiences can fill some of the holes in your soul.

Most people who become addicted to drugs or alcohol have experienced trauma in their lives. Many have experienced deep painful traumas such as violence, sexual assault, abandonment, post-traumatic stress disorder, and more. People do have the capacity to heal from these traumatic experiences, often by reliving the pain, coming to terms with the experience, and reaching a point of acceptance, forgiveness, love, and peace of mind. This healing process can relieve the pain and even fill the hole that was created by the trauma. Individual and group therapies can help people work through these painful experiences. Some experts say that during addiction treatment it may be better not to deal with these most painful traumatic experiences because they will be too much to handle and can lead to relapse. Other experts say that if these experiences are not dealt with during treatment, they will likely just propel the person to relapse at a later time. Both of these outcomes are possible. Meditation can help a person handle the challenge of working through trauma without becoming overwhelmed, when a person is ready to go through this healing experience.

Affirmation

I will mediate daily to help me handle the healing process of my recovery from addiction and trauma.

Thought for Day 77

We are responsible for ourselves—yet we are also responsible for each other.

Before we can accomplish anything in life, we have to meet our own basic needs and take care of ourselves. Waking up with a hangover, using drugs before work, or staying out and drinking until the early morning hours take a toll on our lives. If we don't take care of ourselves, we can't really do much for others. On an airplane, the flight attendant announces that in case of a lack of oxygen, you should place the breathing mask over your mouth before you help others put their masks on. If you can't breathe, function, or survive, you cannot care for other people. So the first thing to do is to take care of your own recovery, take care of yourself. Yet we are also responsible for each other. If we want to survive as a family or as a community, we have to take care of each other. We often have to make compromises to accommodate the needs of others. We have to find a balance between meeting our own needs and meeting the needs of others.

Affirmation

I will make sure that I am taking care of myself while at the same time considering the needs of others in my life.

Thought for Day 78

Sometimes the best thing to do is dance and sing.

Yes, life is serious business. Life can be challenging. Recovery is a tough challenge. Still, we often take life too seriously. Too often we get caught up in the drama at work, at home, or among our friends. We get so overwhelmed by the hundreds and thousands of little details and decisions that seem to strangle our lives. We get stuck in routines, doing the same things day after day. Sometimes we have to let go of our problems, the stress, the guilt, the anger, the sadness, and just have fun. Sometimes for our health and well-being, we have to play hooky—just drop out for the day and play. We have to remind ourselves that life is short. We have to take time to smell the flowers—and take time to connect with the people we love. We have to take time for ourselves to do absolutely nothing. Sometimes we have to dance and sing and play. Sometimes, we simply have to celebrate life.

Affirmation

For a day, for an hour, for a moment, I will listen to the music and let it move my soul.

For many, being alone is a difficult experience.

Why is it so hard sometimes to be alone? Maybe it is just our human nature. When we are young and we are left alone, we become terrified. It is our survival instinct. We cry and scream until someone can hear and take care of us. The need to be with others is naturally and deeply engrained in our souls. At the same time, we cannot avoid being alone during much of our lives. We have to learn how to live with this aloneness. The experience of solitude or being alone is different from loneliness. We have to accept and not fear that we are often alone, even in the midst of people. It is natural. Feel the aloneness. Some people prefer to be alone. This may be because being with others is painful or stressful to them. Yet, others prefer this aloneness because it allows them creative room to be who they are. Whether we like or hate being alone, it's an inevitable experience that we cannot escape.

AFFIRMATION

For a moment in my meditation, I will embrace my aloneness.

Thought for Day 80

We may not like some parts of ourselves, the shortcomings and character defects. But paradoxically, when we accept them, they become less unlikeable.

We all have things that we don't like about ourselves. We wish they would go away. We may try and try, but they remain. Sometimes, we think we have overcome them, but then weeks or months later they return in full force. It can be maddening. It can be discouraging. In fellowship meetings, you may hear others say how their shortcomings keep coming back. Sometimes we pretend they don't exist. But if we are honest with ourselves and face reality, we see that they are there—and they are real. The only thing we can do is to admit that they, too, are a part of ourselves. We have to pay attention to what we don't like about ourselves. We have to be patient, caring, and loving to all parts of who we are, including what we find unlikeable inside us. If we can imagine this unlikable part as a child that is in pain and needs caring, we can begin to accept ourselves for who we are, and then, we may be able to begin to change.

Affirmation

I will focus on acknowledging some aspect of myself that I don't like with acceptance of who I am at this moment.

The place where I am now is exactly where I am supposed to be at this moment.

We often wish we were somewhere else, with someone else, doing something else, and we may have good reasons for wishing so. We may want to set goals and make plans to change our lives so that we can fulfill these wishes. But we cannot snap our fingers and make this happen. There are reasons why we came to the place and situation where we are at this moment, even though sometimes these may not be apparent to us. But here is where we are, and there is nowhere else for us to be at this moment. So live in this moment. Breathe in this moment. Make the best of this moment. Fully experience this moment. Many religions have a prayer that offers thanks to their Higher Power for bringing them to this point in time. Appreciate exactly where you are at this moment, without regret, judgment, or despair—and you will live a deeper, fuller life.

AFFIRMATION

Today I will give thanks for being where I am at this point in time.

Thought for Day 82

Sometimes we have to make radical changes.

Revolutions begin because people feel oppressed. Sometimes you may need a revolution in your life. Sometimes you have to make a radical change in your environment or in the way you deal with others. If you are trapped in a negative relationship, you may need to accept this reality, experience your feelings, and let that experience motivate you to take radical action. You may have to move away from a home or neighborhood, an environment where your using, drinking, and negative behavior took place. If the people you spend your time with do not help you in life and recovery but remain destructive forces, then you need to break away. Accept yourself and your feelings. Yet, at the same time, you may have to reject and change your circumstances if they are oppressive, hurtful, or destructive to the soul of your recovery. Allow yourself to feel the full extent of your situation and feelings. Let this be your guide to changes, inside and out, that you need to make in your life.

Affirmation

Today I will meditate, get in touch with my true feelings, and allow these feelings to guide me in my life.

You cannot force change, but at the same time change takes great courage.

Accept yourself as you are, and recognize the changes that you want to make in your life. Take your time. Make sure of the changes that you want to make. Make a list of them. You often have to experience the full extent of your dissatisfaction to motivate yourself to make real change. Real change is not easy; it takes great courage and an emotional commitment. It took you a long time to become the person who you are today. You will not change overnight. So take your time, meditate, and sit with yourself. Experience who you are, and allow the truth of yourself and your feelings to emerge. You will not have to force action to make changes. Sometimes it will happen naturally. Let others into your life to help sort things out. Suddenly it will be crystal clear to you that you no longer need to be the way you are, and you will be able to change. You may have no other choice once you face the real truth. Accepting the truth will give you the "courage to change the things" you can.

AFFIRMATION

Today I will sit with myself, meditate, and envision my life as it really is and how I would like it to be.

Thought for Day 84

Social change can be led by an individual but will only succeed through the power of a group of people.

If we conclude that we need to change, we will need to seek help to make the changes. Though we have to take the initiative and be the leaders of our own internal change, "the captain of our soul," we still need a sponsor, mentor, or guide to help steer us through rough waters. Once we begin to allow for the possibility of change, we may need help in terms of identifying the specific steps to take. Sponsors are often people in your fellowship with many years of experience in recovery, and they can share with you how to make your progress more effective. They can help you to avoid pitfalls. You may also need the help of another family member, counselor or advisor, or support group to make changes in your relationships, community, or work. Let the power of others and groups help you accomplish your goals.

Affirmation

I will be the leader of the changes I need to make in my life, while at the same time I will accept the support and help I need from others to make these changes.

Vision is important, but it takes blood, sweat, and tears—total commitment—to turn your vision into reality.

Can having a vision or a dream of what we want make it materialize? Can focusing our minds on a specific outcome make it happen? This is not very likely. Definitely having a clear vision and focusing on it can help us to achieve it, but we have to work at it, and sometimes for a very long time before it becomes reality. "Easy does it," people say. "But do it!" Meditating on your vision will help you to stay focused, and may help you to be more disciplined while you work toward your vision. But don't rely on vision alone. Develop your skills. Practice them, and put them to use. Meditation can help you to change and balance personal traits or habits that may interfere with you achieving your vision. It is important to look at yourself as honestly as possible, accept yourself, and when you meditate, you can let those self-defeating habits dissolve as you focus on exhaling and breathing them away. We can break down internal obstacles by focusing on them, but achieving our goals, dreams, and visions will take practice and hard work.

Affirmation

I will meditate, develop my vision, and take the necessary steps to turn my vision into a reality.

Thought for Day 86

Healthy eating and exercise has to be a part of lifelong recovery and living in balance.

It is essential to eat a healthy, balanced diet. Eating lots of fruits, vegetables, and grains is critical to recovery of mind and body. Eat minimal amounts of red meat, sugar, salt, junk food, sodas, and all of the things that you know are unhealthy. It is difficult to maintain a healthy diet and regular exercise in our society. When we go to restaurants, the serving sizes are enormous. We are always encouraged to overeat. We face junk food wherever we look. Try to stock your home with as much healthy food as possible, and try to keep unhealthy junk food out of your home. Drink lots of water. Six to eight eight-ounce glasses a day keeps your system clean. Learn to cook new, healthy meals. It can be fun, and you can experience new tastes and new foods. And don't forget: exercise, walk, run, hike, swim, play, use treadmills and other gym equipment, Rollerblade, skateboard, ski. What do you like to do? Just do it!

Affirmation

Today I will exercise and eat healthy food.

Live a healthy lifestyle.

Living healthy is a way of life. If you eat healthy, get daily exercise and plenty of sleep, practice daily meditation, and care for your mind, then the care of the body and soul can become a deeply engrained lifestyle. It is not just a phase or a fad. Make it a way of life that is nearly as natural as breathing. You will live a richer, fuller, and longer life if you can live a healthy lifestyle. Find joy in your life. Go places and do new things that you never thought of doing before. Do whatever you can to change your past harmful addiction habits and lifestyle. Enjoyment helps to maintain sobriety and prevent relapse. You no longer need to drink, use drugs, smoke, or gamble as the only way to have "fun" in life. The old haunts, streets, neighborhoods, and bars will become boring as you find new sources of joy and meaning and fun. Be brave. Try new things. Find joy in the simple things in life. Meditation breathing exercises can help you to enjoy and appreciate living in the moment, not in the past or the future, but in the *now.*

Affirmation

Today I will renew my commitment to living a healthier, balanced life by meditating or just taking a long serenity walk.

Thought for Day 88

Awaken your mind to your own truth and reality.

Through daily meditation, you can become more aware of what is true and real in your life at this moment. Simply focusing on your breathing—breathing in while repeating the names of the things you want to increase and breathing out while repeating the names of the things you want to reduce in your life—can make a huge difference. You can do this sitting, standing, lying down, in any position, in any place, at any time. Whether for a few minutes or for a half hour, taking time to be totally present in the moment makes you more self-aware. It allows you to experience emotions more fully. It makes you more aware of the holes in your soul and allows you to heal them. It helps you to accept yourself for who you are—good, bad, horrible, and beautiful. It allows you to be more honest with yourself and others. It takes practice and discipline. If you make the commitment, it comes naturally. Make a commitment to life. Make a commitment to your health. Make a commitment to your recovery.

Affirmation

I will meditate on the most important things I want to increase and reduce in my life.

Thought for Day 89

Never stop dancing.

Dance is any movement of the body to a rhythm—any movement and any rhythm. As long as you can move, you can dance. Dance wildly or dance gently, but never stop dancing. Listen to the music within. Feel the music of the city vibrate under your feet. Feel the music of nature. Be at one with the music, and let your body move to it. Rigorous dance is good for your body and good for your soul. Dance alone in a room at home, or dance with someone you love. Dancing can help you to loosen up, free blocked energy or tension, and improve your blood circulation. Dancing can be spiritual, sensual, soothing, or just plain fun. Dancing can be a celebration of life. Close your eyes and just let go. Move your feet, hips, shoulders, arms, hands, and head. Dance until you're exhausted. Dance for a few minutes and feel your mood improve. Dance at any age. At any hour. Dance every day. Dance for life.

Affirmation
Today I will dance. Today I will celebrate life.

Thought for Day 90

Life is a journey. Take the time you need to get to wherever you want to go.

It is important and useful to set goals. However, you do not always have control over how long it will take to meet your goals. "Life" often gets in the way of our goals. We may stumble and fall, or get lost and lose our way. Take time finding your way. Take time to pray and meditate so that you can feel present in the moment and experience the process of change and growth. Experience the journey you take every hour. There is no sense in rushing to get somewhere if you miss all of the beautiful scenes and experiences, including the painful ones, along the way. Fully accept the process as it unfolds and don't worry. You will get there exactly on time, on *your* time. The Twelve Steps and *Living in Balance* teach us to see ourselves, the flaws, the shortcomings, the mistakes made, the holes in our soul, the good with the bad, the victories, the joys, and the strengths inside. A life in recovery is a journey for you to experience fully.

Affirmation

Today I will take my time to experience life fully and to celebrate who I am and where I am at this moment in time.

I hope this book of meditations has been helpful to you as you seek out new paths and experiences in your life.

—JAH

INDEX

Jeffrey A. Hoffman, Ph.D., trained as a clinical psychologist, is coauthor of two addiction treatment programs, *Living in Balance: Moving from a Life of Addiction to a Life of Recovery* and *Adolescent Smoking Cessation Escaping Nicotine and Tobacco (ASCENT)*. He is the founder and CEO of Danya International, Inc., and serves on the boards of several commercial and nonprofit organizations. He is married and has three children and a son-in-law.

Hazelden, a national nonprofit organization founded in 1949, helps people reclaim their lives from the disease of addiction. Built on decades of knowledge and experience, Hazelden offers a comprehensive approach to addiction that addresses the full range of patient, family, and professional needs, including treatment and continuing care for youth and adults, research, higher learning, public education and advocacy, and publishing.

A life of recovery is lived "one day at a time." Hazelden publications, both educational and inspirational, support and strengthen lifelong recovery. In 1954, Hazelden published *Twenty-Four Hours a Day*, the first daily meditation book for recovering alcoholics, and Hazelden continues to publish works to inspire and guide individuals in treatment and recovery, and their loved ones. Professionals who work to prevent and treat addiction also turn to Hazelden for evidence-based curricula, informational materials, and videos for use in schools, treatment programs, and correctional programs.

Through published works, Hazelden extends the reach of hope, encouragement, help, and support to individuals, families, and communities affected by addiction and related issues.